THE BEST OF

Herb Fred, MD

His Insights, Oberserations, and Everyday Reminders

Compiled and edited by
Mark Scheid, PhD

First Edition
Printed in The United States of America

ISBN 978-1-931823-88-3

Front cover design by Hendrik A. van Dijk

Illustrations reproduced with permission of Punch Ltd.
www.punch.co.uk

Designed and Produced by
Kingsley Literary Services
www.kingsleybooks.com

Looking back on my professional career, I see enormous progress in our ability to detect and treat disease. But along with that progress, we have sacrificed to a large extent the very core of doctoring—humanism. We need to recapture the Oslerian spirit and strive diligently to promote and preserve the human element in medicine. To do that, we must have doctors who demonstrate commitment, compassion, candor, and common sense; doctors who can look at, listen to, and talk with their patients; doctors who understand and believe that medicine is a calling, not a business; and doctors who *always* put their patients first.

— HERBERT L. FRED

Herb Fred's Everyday Reminders

1) All patients are interesting, but not all doctors are interested.

2) Anybody can treat, but not anybody can diagnose.

3) Spoon-fed knowledge goes out with the next bowel movement, but self-acquired knowledge sticks.

4) Some doctors make the same mistake over and over again and call it "experience."

5) Common sense is uncommon.

6) The standard of care is substandard.

7) There is no defense against honesty.

8) Never lower your standards, sacrifice your principles, or sell your integrity.

9) Thinking is painful, time-consuming, and difficult. That's why most people avoid it.

10) To learn medicine, all you need is a patient, a medical library, and someone who knows more medicine than you do. Then, as you read about each thing that your patient complains of or exhibits, you will uncover more and more "new" things to read about, your knowledge will grow and grow, but your educational journey will never end.

Contents

INTRODUCTION

Mark Scheid, PhD

A collection of published quotations from a physician might seem unusual to the reader—physicians' writings, after all, are not usually noted for their brevity, clarity, or wit.

Herb's most recent book, *Images of Memorable Cases: 50 Years at the Bedside*, presenting images of 154 clinical cases and inviting the reader to make the appropriate diagnosis, did not offer much in the way of opportunity for these elements of writing... and yet it was nominated for the National Book Award. As far as I know, that represents the first time that a clinical book has been so honored.

This book, on the other hand, is full of examples of what makes Herb Fred's writing unusual: the quotations herein, chosen from more than forty years of medical articles, are clear; they are to the point; and they are memorable.

Most of all—as readers who have been taught by Herb over the years will attest—they convey Herb's distinctive voice: informed, opinionated, penetrating, and most of all, demanding of intellectual clarity and honesty on the part of the physician and intolerant of less than total focus on the welfare of the patient.

In his Foreword, Dr. Denton Cooley invites the reader to "open the book at any page and gain valuable insights." I invite you to read extensively, and experience a short course in the "Herb Fred Medical School," a continuing education credit that will keep you centered on "The Best of Herb Fred."

FOREWORD

Denton Cooley, MD

Surgeon-in-Chief and President Emeritus, Texas Heart Institute

Nationally acclaimed for his leadership in medical education, Dr. Herb Fred has long been devoted to upholding the human element in medicine. During his 50+ years as a full-time medical educator, he has carried on the tradition of the great physician and humanitarian, Dr. William Osler (1849-1919), who emphasized the importance of basic clinical skills practiced at the patient's bedside. Like Dr. Osler, Dr. Fred is also a prolific author, whose works include not only hundreds of medical articles but also three books of essays and an atlas of medical images.

In this—his fifth—book, which comprises quotes from his earlier publications, Dr. Fred laments the prevalence of *hyposkillia* (a deficiency of clinical skills) among today's physicians. As he points out, high-tech—rather than high-touch—medicine is all that many of today's physicians have ever known. They often use sophisticated tests as a first-line approach, ignoring the diagnostic potential of basic bedside methods plus their own five senses and reasoning power. In too many cases, this approach results in mediocrity and "betrayed professionalism."

Dr. Fred's collection of memorable sayings, pithy aphorisms, and clinical pearls offers a welcome antidote to the prevailing medical climate. Like his other books, this one is superbly written, in a lively, conversational style characterized by his trademark wit and humor. Instead of reading it straight through, one can open the book at any page and gain valuable insights.

The author is a wise mentor, whose approach is "old-fashioned" in the best sense. At one point, he asks, "[H]ow many interesting *doctors* do you know?" Anyone who reads this book will agree that Dr. Fred himself is exceptionally interesting and that *The Best of Herb Fred* is very good indeed.

FOREWORD

Ken Sack, MD

Professor of Clinical Medicine, Emeritus,
University of California, San Francisco

During the past 50 years, Herb Fred has been one of the most influential medical educators in this country, perhaps in the world. Yet, many physicians would not recognize his name. Those who would include his many former students and house staff (many of whom have reached positions of national and international prominence), critical readers of the medical literature, members of the prestigious Osler Society, and department chairs in schools of medicine around the country who have had the good fortune of observing him in action as a visiting professor. Included in his numerous honors are a Presidential Citation and the prestigious Distinguished Teacher Award from The American College of Physicians.

Dr. Fred has influenced the practice of medicine even for those who are not aware that he has done so. Many clinical maxims, clinicopathologic correlations, and concepts of treatment are part of our everyday practice of medicine because of his original observations and meticulous descriptions of previously poorly recognized phenomena. His writing is a model of precision and clarity. Small wonder he is a well-known medical editor and has published hundreds of articles, numerous textbook chapters, and several books.

I acknowledge that hyperbole is rampant these days, but if I were to compare Herb Fred with William Osler, I daresay that no one who knows him well would so much as raise an eyebrow. He is one of a handful of profound thinkers in our time, and he has truly been a gift to the medical community. Taking in his pearls of wisdom will leave the reader not only richer for the experience but also more appreciative of the tremendous privilege it is to practice medicine.

FOREWORD

Michel Accad, MD

San Francisco Heart and Vascular Institute,
Seton Medical Center, Daly City, CA

The coat of arms of the Herb Fred Medical Society consists of a caduceus in the center and a letter C at each corner of the blazon. The four C's stand for Commitment, Compassion, Candor, and Common Sense. With this motto, Herb Fred has succeeded in distilling the essential attributes required for excellence in clinical medicine.

Gemologists also use four C's to judge the value of diamond jewelry. To them, the four C's stand for Clarity, Color, Carat, and Cut. It occurred to me that the writings of Dr. Fred fare superbly when appraised according to lapidarian criteria:

—**Clarity:** Herb Fred is a true wordsmith and readers will experience his prose to be free of any superfluous word or ambiguity. "Better clear than clever," he once taught me. He is a master at making a point with forceful limpidity.

—**Color:** Dr. Fred's jocularity is vivid and irresistible. A great medical aphorist, he can concoct a profound remark into a colorful and memorable zinger, in the manner of Mark Twain or Yogi Berra, yet so unique that his notorious teaching maxims are fondly recalled by his former students as "Fredisms."

—**Carat (weight):** Herb Fred's essays do not delve in trivialities. The delivery may be light but the underlying message is hefty: medicine has lost its way. Dr. Fred points to the atrophy of clinical skills, the over-reliance on technology, the "sagging professionalism," and the increasingly pervasive dishonesty in medicine. These are matters of utmost importance for doctors, patients, and society at large. His observations are grave but he provides physicians with the antidote for the malady: apply the four C's every day and always serve the patient first.

—**Cut:** A diamond cutter aims for specific cutting angles to create edges that brilliantly reflect and refract light. With angles of honesty, intelligence, perspicacity, wit, and wisdom, Herb Fred's writings reflect and refract the truth with sparkle and luminosity.

Mark Scheid has selected from Dr. Fred's *corpus* the very finest gems. They are carefully displayed and organized by theme, and also include a glossary of clinical pearls. Open the book, be dazzled and enlightened!

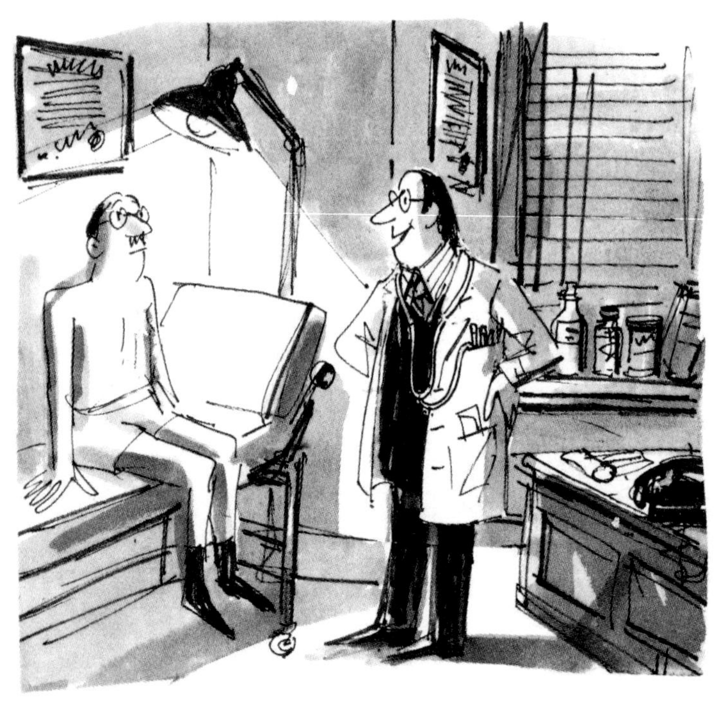

"You're in pretty good shape. You should stand up to hospital treatment."

Chapter One: Life Lessons

Stupidity is essentially God-given; ignorance is clearly man-made. We are only as ignorant as we choose to be.[1]

Crowded restaurants are common. How common are crowded libraries? [2]

Why all this fuss about words? Because words form language, language enables communication, and communication is our link with each other. Without communication, marriages fail, businesses fold, and education flounders.[3]

Regular exercise, regardless of its type, induces a sense of well-being that only those "who have been there" can truly appreciate. Admittedly, millions of people feel fine without any sort of planned physical activity. They would feel better, however, if they adopted an exercise program.[4]

To rise above the norm of mediocrity, one must strive diligently for excellence.[5]

We tend to take our five senses for granted, at least until one of them gets sick. When that happens, the victim has what I call the "sick sense syndrome." It can affect our sense of sight, hearing, touch, taste, or smell.

But the most common type of sensory failure—the one that harms all of us the most—is failure to use our *common* sense. I call that the "sick sixth sense syndrome." [6]

Think for yourself, organize your thoughts carefully, then convey them clearly, succinctly, emphatically, and with honesty. When we do that, we do more than separate shit from shinola. We become leaders, not followers; and we rise above the norm of mediocrity.[7]

If you can't write legibly, print.[8]

The best way to avoid illness and protect against premature coronary artery disease is to bypass smoking, overeating, and inactivity—the kind of triple bypass therapy all of us can afford. [9]

There is more to an education than academics.[10]

We always find time to eat. Yet how often do we find time to feast on books and other material outside our line of work? [11]

Death can bring happiness as well as sorrow, togetherness as well as loneliness, and tranquility as well as turmoil. And the way we die, like the way we live, can teach much and inspire many.[12]

Experts can be wrong.[13]

Achieving and maintaining a thin body or a fat mind necessitate desire, discipline, and dedication. For most of us, a thin body means decreasing our food intake and increasing our physical activity. For *all* of us, however, a fat mind means a diet rich in intellectual calories, devoured regularly and assimilated through repeated mental gymnastics.[11]

Maxwell Wintrobe once wrote, "... many look, but few see." Today, few see because few look.[14]

One sees what one looks *for,* not what one looks *at.*[15]

In today's world, "four-letter word" is an imprecise term with a precise connotation. Everybody knows that it's the nice way of referring to not-so-nice words. And just about everybody hears, sees, says, or thinks four-letter words daily.

But today's world would be better off if we spent less time broadcasting four-letter words and more time exchanging "four-word letters." After all, nobody doesn't like a "thank you very much."[16]

Many careers reflect ascent by assent.[17]

Today's truths are tomorrow's fallacies.[18]

Compassion can develop early if we have the right role models. When we witness compassion, we can give it more easily; but we cannot feel its full significance until we receive it when we need it. Though most physicians have compassion, many are unable to show it.

Common sense, in contrast to book sense, is inherent. We either have it or we don't. And not using it is worse than not having it.

Lastly, wisdom: If it comes at all, it comes with age.[19]

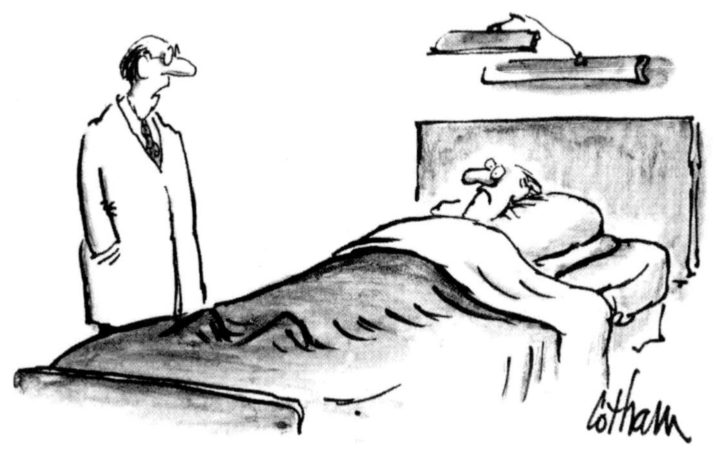

"You put on a white coat and everyone assumes you're a doctor."

Chapter Two: On Medical Education

Part A: On Teaching

Whatever the future brings, we must always view medicine as a calling, not a business, and hold fast to the patient-oriented traditions that have sustained our profession throughout its history.[20]

American medical schools have always valued research over teaching. This stance had little detrimental effect on medical education for most of the past century. But now, the ever-increasing emphasis on technology, the shrinking of government funding of medical services, and the devastating impact of managed care have delivered a serious blow to clinical teaching. Medical schools are so strapped for money these days that they force the clinical faculty to spend progressively more time caring for patients who can pay their bills and progressively less time caring for medical students and house officers. Consequently, trainees are left to fend for themselves in the quest for competency, unaware of how much better their lot could be and should be.

At present, house officers learn clinical medicine primarily from each other, rather than from veteran clinicians. Students, in turn, learn clinical medicine primarily from house officers who are several years their senior but are not necessarily more knowledgeable or competent. This arrangement had merit many years ago when residencies, in contrast to internships, were reserved for the elite. In those days, acceptance into a residency provided no guarantee of completing it. And since most training programs had a pyramid structure, attrition always occurred: only the best residents remained. From that group, one resident ultimately became the chief resident, who also served as chief assistant to the departmental chair.

Today, residency positions are much more numerous and much easier to obtain. And because the pyramid structure is largely a relic of the past, the relative number of weak residents has risen. In many ways, therefore, we now have a see-one, do-one, teach-one system that fosters mediocrity, stifles individuality, promotes incompetence, and permits—if not encourages—dishonesty.[21]

Learning the best way to learn medicine is something many physicians never learn.[5]

"Idiopathic" is a pseudoscientific and quasi-intellectual way of saying "I don't know." But since most doctors have difficulty saying "I don't know," the tag "idiopathic" is destined to remain forever ensconced in the medical lingo. This is unfortunate, because our habit of substituting labels for diagnoses all too frequently lulls us into diagnostic complacency and dulls any further cerebration. The patient, in turn, suffers the consequences. To combat this ongoing danger, I have coined the term *idiotopathic.* It looks and sounds like *idiopathic,* but it makes us more mindful of our ignorance—while still satisfying our penchant for labels.[22]

Throughout high school, college, and medical school, I thought that learning depended on having a good teacher. When I was an intern, however, I began to realize that the most active role in my education belonged to me. Later, when I myself became a teacher, I realized that a good teacher teaches by promoting learning; and he promotes learning primarily by the questions he asks, not by the answers he gives. Repeated exposure to this Socratic method teaches the student the types of questions to ask himself and when to ask them. From then on he learns most and best from one teacher—himself.[23]

Arrogance among physicians is common. But our arrogance often is a front for ignorance and insecurity and can crumble as knowledge builds. We can also fight any godlike tendencies with an "anti-deiotic"—a mixture of humility and honesty.[5]

Categorizing patients as interesting—or not interesting—is a habit that all physicians have. It starts in medical school, reaches a peak during postgraduate training, and persists to varying degrees throughout our professional careers. In fact, it becomes so much a part of us that we rarely give it any thought. We should.

Like beauty, the interesting patient is in the eye of the beholder. A woman with argyria, for example, would be interesting to a dermatologist but not necessarily to an orthopedic surgeon. Similarly, a man with a dissecting aneurysm of the aorta would be interesting to a cardiologist but perhaps not to a psychiatrist. And a big liver would be more interesting to a medical student who had never felt one than to a veteran clinician who had felt hundreds. Nevertheless, any patient can be interesting if the doctor is interested.

Incidentally, how many interesting *doctors* do you know?[24]

Mandated work-hour limits across all teaching programs have dealt a serious blow to medical education. I have previously argued that cutting back on training hours adversely affects patient care and promotes physician incompetence. Such cutbacks, in fact, may ultimately necessitate prolongation of training in some specialties.[25]

Courses in physical diagnosis are frequently disjointed, inserted piecemeal into already crowded curricula, and taught by residents, fellows, and junior faculty members. One medical resident told me that in his physical diagnosis course, the only exposure he had to the optic fundus was a lecture by an ophthalmologist who showed slides but gave no hands-on instruction. Other residents told me that during their third and fourth years in medical school, there was no organized attempt to help them acquire skills in using the ophthalmoscope. No wonder they use it so sparingly now.[14]

Today, in the era of high-tech medicine, we need to remember the value of a carefully documented medical history, which includes attention to previous medical records. If we forget, the consequences will be costly—more ill-advised procedures, higher medical bills, and greater patient suffering.[26]

Studies indicate that between 27% and 58% of students cheat at least once in medical school, that those who cheat are likely to be dishonest when providing patient care during their clerkships, and that the number of students who cheat increases from the freshman to the senior year.

I firmly believe that there is no place in medicine for cheaters or liars. In today's permissive culture, however, automatic expulsion of such miscreants—the rule when I was in training—no longer occurs, and most of these guilty students (and house officers) ultimately enter private practice or remain in academic medicine. Not surprisingly, this unprofessional behavior in medical school correlates strongly with subsequent disciplinary action by state medical boards.[27]

Not all hospitalized patients need their temperature, pulse, respiration, and blood pressure checked every six to eight hours. But such orders are routine virtually everywhere. Additionally, not all patients with fever and cough need their sputum stained and cultured for acid-fast and fungal organisms. But orders to that effect are disappointingly common, especially in teaching hospitals.[8]

From its roots as a patient-centered, education-oriented year of learning, the medical internship has evolved into a laboratory-centered, algorithm-oriented, technology-driven, computer-dependent, Internet-based, "treat first, diagnose later" training program. Consequently, we are exchanging sleep-deprived healers for a cadre of wide-awake technicians who cannot take an adequate medical history, cannot perform a reliable physical examination, cannot critically assess information they gather, cannot create a sound management plan, have little reasoning power, and communicate poorly.[20]

To me, the most common, and yet most subtle expression of betrayed professionalism is serving ourselves before serving our patients. By doing so, we sacrifice the very core of good doctoring—humanism. And as a result, the patient-physician bond becomes weakened—or never even forms.

Old-fashioned hard work, devotion to duty, and pursuit of excellence have taken a back seat to an emphasis on limited work hours and quests for financial and other types of personal gains. As a result, people at all levels—including many physicians—are satisfied with mediocrity. In fact, mediocrity has become the standard. Given this environment, no wonder our professionalism sags.

Can we remedy our sagging professionalism? Only insofar as we are willing to be role models of integrity and honesty for each other. Only if we show commitment, compassion, competence, candor, and common sense. Only if we understand and believe that medicine is a calling, not a business. Only if we strive diligently to restore, preserve, and promote the human element in medicine. Only if we look at, listen to, and talk with our patients, working as hard and as long as it takes to ensure their welfare. Only if we always put our patients first.[28]

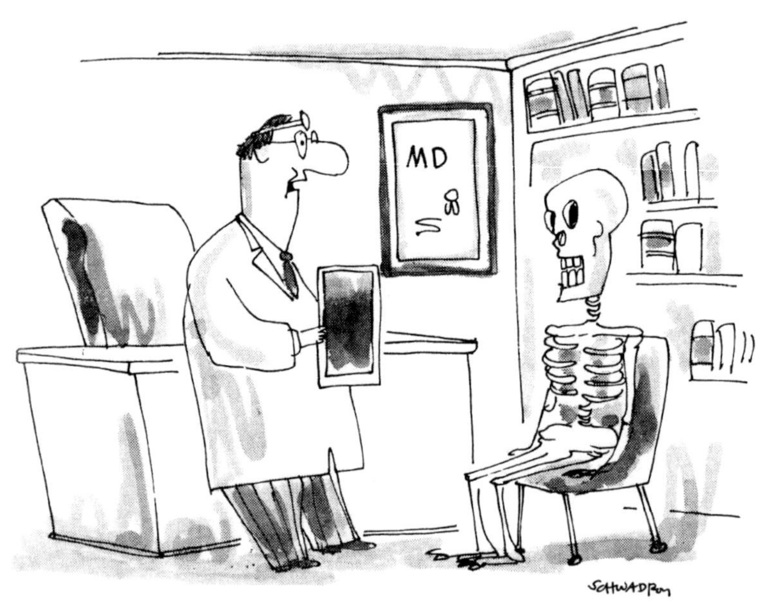

"Your X-rays came back. But they didn't tell us anything we didn't already know."

PART B: ON DIAGNOSIS

The course in physical diagnosis at most American medical schools today is woefully inadequate. Many of these courses consist mainly, if not totally, of lectures. And if any hands-on teaching occurs, house officers (even at times senior students or nurses) typically do it.[29]

For me, the MD after my name means more than "medical doctor." It means "making decisions." And making correct medical decisions requires an ability to distinguish between cause and coincidence. That ability, in turn, requires knowledge of the pathogenesis and natural history of diseases.[30]

John Milton (1608-1674), generally regarded as the greatest poet of his time, began losing his eyesight in 1644. By 1652, Milton had become totally blind, after which he wrote the sonnet, "On His Blindness." The last line of that sonnet, *"They also serve who only stand and wait,"* expresses Milton's belief that blindness does not preclude service to one's God. For me, however, those words are a perfect mnemonic for remembering that disciplined, thoughtful observation is at times the best way to serve our patients. Accordingly, in 1978, I named that approach, "Milton's Law."

Willie Sutton (1901-1980) was well-known for his ingenuity in robbing banks and escaping from prisons. One day, the story goes, he was asked why he robbed banks. Reportedly, he answered, "Because that's where the money is." His logic spurred William Dock (1898-1990), an internationally prominent internist and cardiologist, to coin "Sutton's Law"—go straight to where the diagnosis is. Sutton's Law gained immediate popularity because it reminded physicians to bypass unnecessary, inconclusive, and often expensive studies.

In contrast, Milton's Law never caught on. And unfortunately, with the advent of high-tech diagnostic methods such as magnetic resonance imaging and computed tomography, Sutton's Law gradually disappeared from the medical literature and is rarely remembered today.

Both laws deserve to be resurrected: the words of a master poet pleading for careful, thought-filled inaction and the logic of a master criminal advocating specific, well-directed action. Proper blending of these concepts defines the art of medicine: "know what to do and when to do it." I call that Mutton's Law! [31]

We need more teachers who learned to make diagnoses by understanding the pathophysiology, clinical features, and natural history of diseases. They know what tests, if any, to order, when to order them, and how to interpret them. And they use advanced technology to *verify* rather than to *formulate* their clinical impressions.

These are the teachers who truly comprehend the value of a good medical history, the rewards of a pertinent physical examination, and the power of knowing how to think. These are the teachers who still routinely use the stethoscope, not an echocardiogram, to detect valvular heart disease; who use the ophthalmoscope, not magnetic resonance imaging, to detect intracranial hypertension; who use their eyes, not a blood gas apparatus, to detect cyanosis; who use their hands, not computed tomography, to detect splenomegaly; and who use their brain and their heart, not a horde of consultants, to manage their patients.

And these are the teachers who don't order expensive, state-of-the-art studies when cheaper, conventional tests supply the same information; who don't administer a slew of medications in an effort to alleviate every possible ill; who appreciate that doing nothing is, at times, doing a lot; and who realize that many patients get well despite what we do, not because of what we do.

Unfortunately, these necessary role models are a vanishing species. Most of them have died or retired, and those who still have regular contact with medical students and house officers are too few to stem the tide of technologic tenesmus.[32]

Doctors and trains have several things in common. Both serve the public, both have tight schedules, both run for hours without stopping, and both frequently arrive late. Most important, both may get derailed—one mechanically, the other diagnostically—particularly when they go too fast or fail to heed warning signals.

Derailed trains can't think themselves back on track. Derailed doctors can.[33]

It doesn't matter so much in CPCs if the diagnosis is wrong as long as the *approach* to the diagnosis is right. Getting the wrong diagnosis for the right reasons is better than getting the right diagnosis for the wrong reasons. Failure to understand or accept this principle greatly reduces the benefits of the CPC.

Diseases such as liver abscess, pancreatic carcinoma, and subdural hematoma—frequent culprits in CPCs of yesteryear—rarely qualify for CPCs today. Moreover, in years past, the CPC protocol primarily emphasized the patient's medical history, physical examination, and hospital course. Nowadays, laboratory data take center stage.

The main participants in CPCs have also changed. For many years, the same clinician and pathologist usually conducted the conferences, no matter what disease the patient had. These days, the clinician and pathologist vary according to the subspecialty into which the case fits.

The glory days of the CPC appear to be over—master clinicians are almost extinct, bedside skills are neither fashionable nor commonly sought, treatment has overtaken diagnosis as a priority in medical education, and the medical profession has become more of a business than a calling.

Nevertheless, until doctors are no longer necessary for health care, I believe that a well-planned CPC will continue to be a worthwhile educational activity. After all, where else can we exercise an important part of our body without buying expensive equipment, risking serious injury, or upsetting our spouse?[34]

Afraid of missing the diagnosis, many physicians order a multitude of tests and an army of consultants. This practice is haphazard, time-consuming, unduly expensive, and occasionally dangerous.[8]

Life-saving treatment can be life-threatening if the diagnosis is wrong.[35]

Information from previous medical records can be crucial, both to patient care and to physician education. Yet, on teaching rounds these days, I find that such records get little more than lip service. House officers frequently don't try to obtain them, rarely appreciate the need to get them promptly, and generally show limited ability to scrutinize them effectively once in hand. And these records typically are missing at case presentations.

The genesis of this problem seems clear: Medicine has moved from "high touch" to "high tech," and medical education has shifted its focus accordingly. As a consequence, today's trainees, many of their teachers, and many private practitioners are becoming prisoners of the laboratory, deprived of the joy and satisfaction of using one's mind and five senses to make diagnoses. Thus, they often overlook an integral part of the medical history—the patient's medical records.[26]

The good doctor knows what to do and when to do it. But the very good doctor knows what not to do and when not to do it.[36]

Feeling a big gallbladder at the bedside should be more gratifying than finding it first by ultrasonography, computerized tomographic scanning, or magnetic resonance imaging. Which brings me to this question: Would you know a gallbladder if you felt one? [37]

Put your thoughts in order before you order.[8]

The right approach to a diagnostic problem can sometimes uncover an answer that had not been considered.[13]

When the right diagnostic bell doesn't ring, you may be in the wrong belfry.[38]

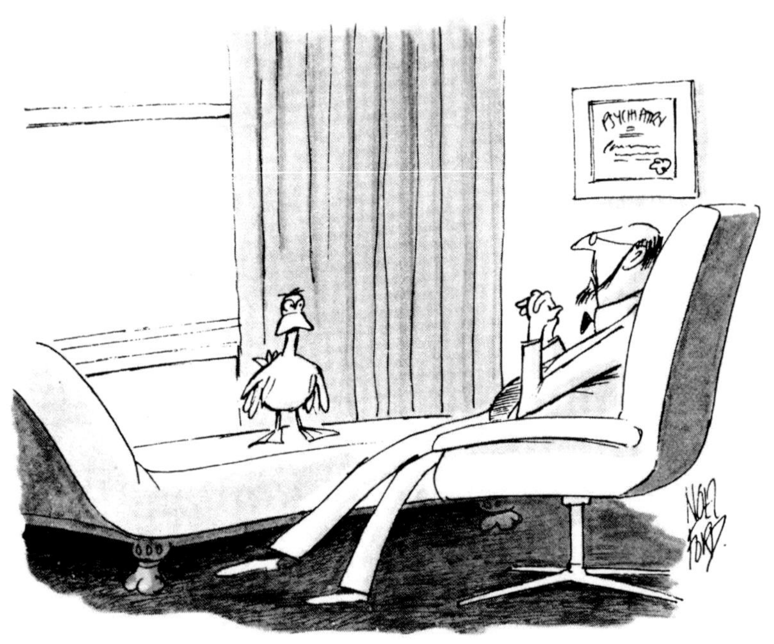

"There's nothing I can do for you—you <u>*are*</u> *a duck."*

Part C: On Technology

Knowing that you *know* is just as important as knowing that you *don't* know. For example, if you see an animal that has webbed feet and feathers, lives in and around water, and goes "quack-quack," you *know* it's a duck. And you don't have to rely on tests and consultants to rule out a chicken, a fish, or a rabbit.[39]

Doctors nowadays rely heavily on instruments other than their eyes and brains to help them see what they look at. One such instrument is "the scope," of which there are many.

Of the scopes currently available, the oldest and most reliable is the retrospectoscope. It is our best teaching instrument.

Much more difficult to master than the retrospectoscope is the prospectoscope. Clarity and correctness of vision through *this* instrument are directly proportional to the competence of the user.

Once we are proficient in using both the retrospectoscope and the prospectoscope, we are ready to use the perspectoscope—the scope that all patients deserve. This scope brings everything into perspective and keeps it there.[40]

"Technologic tenesmus," the uncontrollable urge to rely on sophisticated medical gadgetry for diagnoses,... pervades our profession and has reached epidemic proportions. It is insidious in onset, highly contagious, and rapidly addictive. All of us are endangered, particularly the ill-trained or ill-informed, and those looking for shortcuts, fearing litigation, or lacking in self-confidence. Unaware of their affliction, the victims become tools of the laboratory—shackled to the routine of using advanced technology to *formulate* rather than to *verify* their clinical impressions.[32]

Formerly, we put our thoughts in order before we ordered tests; now we order tests to generate our thoughts.[41]

With so many sophisticated tests and procedures at our disposal, we have fallen in love with numbers and have unwittingly acquired a laboratory-oriented rather than a patient-oriented mind-set. Inadequate training, insufficient clinical experience, and plain old ignorance undoubtedly contribute to this behavior.[42]

CT cannot substitute for examining the spinal fluid. Each year, for example, I come across patients in whom the cranial CT is normal but the lumbar puncture yields findings diagnostic of a specific disorder.

We should remember, too, that CT cannot provide histologic evidence. Yet, I continue to see CT reports—especially when the head is scanned—that conclude with precise diagnoses, such as "metastases," "infarct," and "toxoplasmosis." Reports of this sort do more to boost tunnel vision than to enhance patient care.[36]

When the CT scanner breaks down or is otherwise unavailable, patient-oriented activities largely come to a halt. I have observed this phenomenon on several occasions and consider it a sad reflection of today's practice of medicine.[21]

Nearly all of today's teachers of medicine received their training after the early 1970s—the time when modern medical technology began to burgeon. High-tech medicine is all they've ever seen, all they know, and, therefore, all they know to teach. Through no fault of their own, they have no real sense of high-touch medicine: medicine based on a carefully constructed medical history coupled with a pertinent physical examination and critical assessment of the information obtained therefrom.[21]

Computed tomography is magnificent, but it cannot detect hysteria.[21]

If more doctors today practiced medicine the old-fashioned way, our profession might regain some of the nobility and respect it once enjoyed.[34]

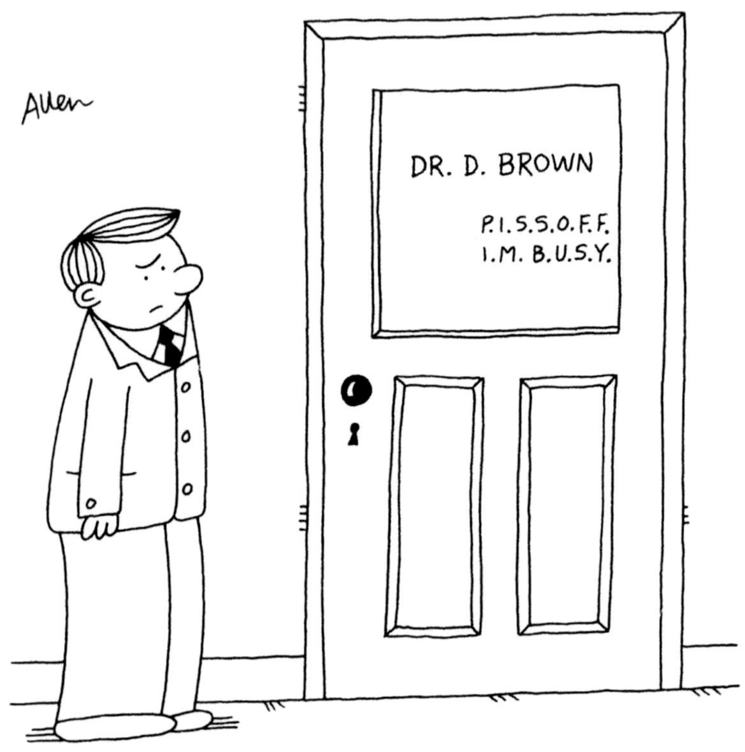
Allen
DR. D. BROWN
P.I.S.S.O.F.F.
I.M. B.U.S.Y.

Part D: Medical Literature and Medical Communication

"Scholarly," like beauty, is in the eye of the beholder. *Scholarly* is also a buzzword, one that we wield to impress our subordinates and to compliment or denigrate the work of our colleagues. And, in the publishing game, this role of "scholarly" can sink, or save, a manuscript.[43]

I believe that being a competent doctor requires more than having the latest scientific facts. I also believe that some of the most rewarding information in medical journals has little to do with science per se.[44]

In academia, we usually embrace whatever the professor says or whatever the textbook or medical journal declares. We don't always realize or remember that another professor, another journal, or another text may put an entirely different spin on the same subject. History, both medical and general, is filled with stories of individuals who tried to introduce new ideas but couldn't penetrate the party line. This barrier continues to produce blind acquiescence and stifled innovation.[5]

Some journal editors and commercial publishers—even some university presses—opt for bulk over brevity, size over substance, matter over mind. If everyone used this logic, however, manuscripts without padding and puffery wouldn't qualify as "scholarly" and might not merit publication. And the Ten Commandments, Declaration of Independence, and Gettysburg Address—each pithy, perspicuous, and profound—might never have made it into print.[43]

Dishonesty in medical research boils down to 2 basic kinds of participants: 1) ambitious investigators whose quest for fame and glory overshadows whatever integrity they might have, and 2) financially motivated drug companies that spare nothing in their attempts to capture a dominant share of the pharmaceutical market.[27]

Because of their ambiguity, abbreviations in medicine can be dangerous. If they go unquestioned, particularly in doctors' orders and prescriptions, the patient may get the wrong test or the wrong medication, with devastating results.[45]

TIA is a TIA—Treacherously Inadequate Acronym.[46]

Improper use of acronyms has become a nemesis. Hence, our term "acronymesis"…

Editors need to Concentrate On Nixing This Rarely Obvious Lingo (CONTROL), and authors need to remember that good Communicators Resist Acronymic Proliferation (CRAP).[47]

To most English-speaking humans on this planet, BM is short for bowel movement. Yet many physicians seem oblivious to this fact and use BM to mean black male. (How would you like to be called a BM?) Depending on one's frame of reference, however, BM also represents bone marrow, basement membrane, basal metabolism, body mass, breast milk, blood monocyte, buccal mass, bachelor of medicine, bacterial meningitis, betamethasone, and biomedical.

When reading patients' charts, I commonly find abbreviations that I have never seen before and cannot for the life of me decipher. One in particular really caught my attention—LGFTD. Who would ever have guessed that LGFTD stands for "Looks good from the door."

Will the pandemic of abbreviations in medicine ever end? Not unless we learn to value clarity and precision over self-serving, thoughtless shortcuts. And not until we concede that abbreviations do nothing for our patients except place them at risk—emotionally, physically, and financially.[48]

Remember, the only person who invariably knows what an abbreviation stands for is the one who uses it. [8]

Fabricating or manipulating data is the most egregious form of dishonesty in the medical literature. In most cases, however, its detection is virtually impossible. So caveat lector—let the reader beware! [27]

"To my knowledge" is a phrase whose appearance in current medical literature has reached epidemic proportions. Why? Does any writer know everything about his topic? Does the ploy shield the author from criticism and excuse him from more work? Does the device improve a manuscript's clarity, ensure its validity, or strengthen its message? Does the tactic satisfy discerning readers?

No. Well, perhaps not. At least, not to my knowledge! [49]

Recommended reading for students and practitioners of medicine does not ordinarily include references to the obligations of our profession, to our own frailties, to speculative thinking, or to medical history. It should! [44]

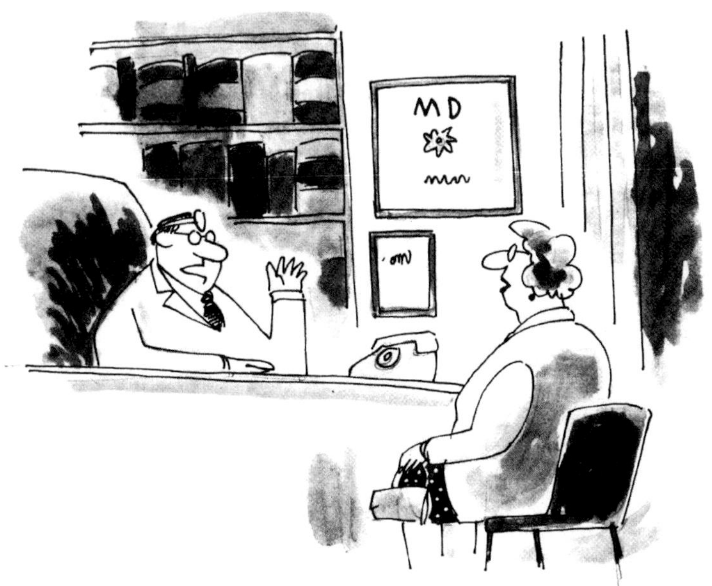

"Woah! Slow down, Mrs Marney. Please keep in mind I have to translate all your laymen's terms into medical gobbledygook."

Chapter Three: On the Practice of Medicine

Herd mentality—the unwillingness or inability to think for one's self—permeates our profession. Boosted by the medical technology at our disposal these days, this mental inertia adversely affects all aspects of patient care, especially proper decision-making and effective communication. This inertia also dampens requisite curiosity and impedes self-education. And if it continues at its current pace, the core values of our profession—displaying humanism, striving for excellence, being honest, embracing sacrifice, promoting skepticism, avoiding arrogance, and always putting the patient first—seem destined for oblivion.[50]

Treat your patient, not yourself.[8]

A serious malady undermines our profession. I call it diagnostic and therapeutic tenesmus. It typically strikes house officers and young practitioners, but even experienced physicians are afflicted. The victims have an uncontrollable urge to diagnose and treat. Without proper attention to the clinical picture, they order myriad tests and prescribe a multitude of drugs, hoping to detect and alleviate every possible ill. Their approach is haphazard, time-consuming, unduly expensive, and sometimes dangerous.[51]

Whether chest pain is typical or not depends primarily on one's perception of "typical." Such perception, in turn, depends on one's depth of medical knowledge and the time spent evaluating the patient. Remember that in the individual case, manifestations of any disease fall somewhere on a bell-shaped curve. Unless we are familiar with the manifestations at either end of the curve, we will interpret them as atypical even though they are, in fact, typical. Stated another way, the pain may be truly atypical of the disease we are thinking of (for example, angina pectoris) but clearly typical of one we aren't thinking of (pericardial fat pad necrosis). Furthermore, in the zeal to prove our initial impression, we may set in motion a "fruitless search for infallibility," resulting in a host of ill-directed, expensive, time-consuming, and sometimes dangerous studies.

Delivering good health care these days is hard enough without using Humpty-Dumpty terminology. Instead of "atypical chest pain," I recommend substituting "chest pain, ? cause" or "unexplained chest pain." Doing so would reduce the risk of miscommunication, remind us of our ignorance, stimulate us to think, and keep us honest with ourselves and our patients.[52]

For us oldies in medicine, doing nothing means doing a lot. It means not ordering expensive, state-of-the-art studies when cheaper, conventional tests would supply the same information. It means not administering a slew of medications in an attempt to alleviate every possible ill. It means not requesting numerous consultations just because the diagnosis is not immediately obvious. It means appreciating the opportunities to learn the natural history of disease. It means realizing that many patients get well in spite of what we do, not because of what we do.[53]

Good patient rapport is the best protection against lawsuits.[51]

For me, MD has a special meaning: *Making Decisions.* Indeed, making medical decisions is what we physicians are licensed and obligated to do. Yet too often we decide not to decide. We shun this basic responsibility and delegate it to a committee of colleagues, to the patient, or to the patient's family.

Making correct decisions in medicine requires continually updated scientific knowledge and a skillfully selected data base. But it takes candor and courage, too.

Wear MD legitimately. *Make Decisions!* [54]

An algorithm is a tool that physicians have borrowed from mathematicians to solve diagnostic (and sometimes therapeutic) problems. Therein lies my first objection to the use of algorithms in medical practice. Mathematicians manage numbers. Physicians manage patients. Sadly, however, more and more physicians are managing numbers rather than the patients who have those numbers. And algorithms undoubtedly contribute to this deplorable trend.

Another drawback of algorithms is their all-too-frequent complexity. On occasion, I see algorithms that occupy an entire printed page. They have so many steps with so many arrows pointing in so many directions that I ultimately give up trying to figure everything out.

Do algorithms leave room for clinical judgment and compassion? No.

Do algorithms take into account the wide variation in disease manifestations and in patient responses? Certainly not.

Do algorithms improve the patient-doctor relationship? No, they replace it—the doctor interacts with the algorithm, not the patient.

I suggest that we give algorithms back to the mathematicians—and focus instead on expanding our medical knowledge, honing our bedside skills, strengthening our clinical judgment, and displaying compassion. If we do, our patients will be the better for it. [55]

The fact is, we doctors regularly invade our patients in one way or another, though we don't always perceive it as such. We invade their privacy by the medical histories we take and the physical examinations we do. We puncture their skin to draw blood. We stick catheters into their bladders, put tubes down their throats, place speculums in their vaginas, and insert scopes up their rectums. And most of what we do invades their pocketbooks. [56]

A good doctor blends compassion with candor, book sense with common sense. He strives diligently to maintain perspective, focusing on the patient, not the disease. He always finds time to listen to those seeking his help; perceives more than just their words; and talks with, not to, them in an easily understood way. He thinks for himself and makes his own decisions. He relies chiefly on his mind and five senses for diagnoses; knows the indications for and limitations of laboratory procedures; and uses tests and consultants to verify, not formulate, his clinical impressions. He respects and appreciates nurses, technicians, and other members of the health-care team. And, cognizant of his own fallibility, he is never afraid to say, "I don't know."[57]

Legitimate medical practice has its gimmicks—technologically advanced, scientifically sound procedures *misused* by physicians who are ill-trained, ill-informed, lacking in self-confidence, looking for short-cuts, fearful of litigation, or just plain greedy. Such gimmicks are used without regard for their indications or limitations and take precedence over diagnostic methods that are simpler, less expensive, and equally effective.

Gimmicks have no judgment or common sense, show no compassion or understanding, and never look at or listen to the patient. A good doctor does.[58]

Overreliance on modern technology is undermining the physician's use of his mind and five senses for diagnoses. Jumping from the patient's chief complaint to a host of tests and procedures is commonplace. And when that approach does not work, the physician simply orders more tests or seeks consultation. This malady of practice is making the skilled clinical diagnostician a vanishing species. It is taking much of the fun and challenge out of medicine. It is depersonalizing the doctor-patient relationship. Even worse, it threatens the individuality of patient care.[58]

Nowadays, calling in a consultant all too frequently is a way for physicians to save time and thought, protect themselves against malpractice suits, or repay colleagues for previous favors. Consequently, the procedure has lost the planning, formality, and professionalism it once had.[59]

Like football coaches, we physicians try to call the right play at the right time. To do so, we need what I call "press box vision"—a view of the situation in perspective. Without press box vision, the coach and his team may lose. But football is just a game. Practicing medicine isn't.[60]

Physicians do not have the privilege of shirking responsibility.[61]

The care that any hospitalized patient receives—be it good or otherwise—ultimately depends on what the doctor orders, how those orders are interpreted, and when and how they are implemented. Yet, formal instruction in order-writing has never been part of the medical school curriculum and probably never will be. Furthermore, the medical literature and standard medical textbooks devote little attention to the subject. And few attending physicians regularly critique house officers' orders. Consequently, medical students and house officers "learn" order-writing from each other—the "see-one, do-one, teach-one" method.[8]

Many nurses are reluctant to seek clarification of an order because the physician's response all too frequently is abusive (e.g., "Can't you read?" or "Don't bother me, I'm busy" or something even more insulting). As a result, the order may be carried out incorrectly—or not at all. So, if the nurse questions you, be appreciative, and respond accordingly.[8]

"Please" and "thank you" are words that rarely find their way onto the doctor's order sheet. But when they do, they do wonders for the nurse-doctor relationship—which in turn benefits the patient. 8

Surely each of us can recall (with regrets) clinical situations in which we were quick to act and slow to think. Perhaps Alexander Pope had us in mind when he wrote, "Fools rush in where angels fear to tread." 35

Dishonesty in medical practice takes many forms, virtually all of which stem from the same cause—serving one's self before serving one's patients. A prime example is shirking responsibility (that is, failure to take charge). In such cases, the attending physician—faced with a busy schedule and fearful of being sued for missing something—orders myriad tests and prescribes a multitude of drugs, hoping thereby to detect and alleviate every conceivable ill. If the patient's condition fails to improve or a test result is abnormal, the attending physician defers to an army of consultants who march in and take over, each managing a part of the body but no one managing the whole.

A cascade of ill-advised activities ensues—more consultations, inappropriate testing, over-prescribing of medications, uncalled-for procedures, needlessly prolonged hospitalizations, and unnecessary office visits. This process continues until a definitive diagnosis surfaces, the patient's complaints subside, the patient or the patient's family intervenes, or the patient dies. Meanwhile, the attending physician simply watches the medical merry-go-round. 27

I remember when—

- Consultants rendered opinions, not mandates.
- Health insurance was affordable and easy to get.

- Medical malpractice suits were virtually unheard of, and lawyers were physicians' friends.
- Taking a good medical history and doing a careful physical examination were coveted skills.
- An ECHO was something you might hear after shouting in a canyon, MRI referred to moderate renal insufficiency, and a CAT scan meant stealing a glimpse of your feline pet.

I remember when Medicine was a highly respected calling, the noblest of professions.[62]

Good care for some patients calls for the same degree of circumspection required when handling a rattlesnake. Failure to heed this principle does a disservice to the patient and invites trouble for the physician. The trick, therefore, is to recognize the diverse situations in which such circumspection is paramount.[35]

Health care delivery in America today is fragmented, impersonal, costly, and marred by adverse events. Patients, however, aren't the only ones to bear the brunt. Doctors who render the care, including those of us in medical research and education, are also adversely affected. We have lost much of our autonomy, have seen our prestige plummet, and find ourselves marching to bureaucratic drummers. Frustration, disappointment, and to some extent frank disgust permeate our ranks.[25]

From my observations, I believe that most doctors work hard and mean well. But I also believe that doctors are a lot like elephants: we tend to follow the herd rather than think for ourselves. This mental inertia undermines patient care, dulls intellectual curiosity, impedes self-education, hinders decision making, and cripples effective communication. It is more common among doctors than alcoholism or drug abuse and is potentially more devastating to society. Yet it gets almost no attention.[63]

I call this malady *hyposkillia*—deficiency of clinical skills. By definition, those afflicted are ill-equipped to render good patient care. Yet, residency training programs across the country are graduating a growing number of these "hyposkilliacs"—physicians who cannot take an adequate medical history, cannot perform a reliable physical examination, cannot critically assess the information they gather, cannot create a sound management plan, have little reasoning power, and communicate poorly. Moreover, they rarely spend enough time to know their patients "through and through." And because they are quick to treat everybody, they learn nothing about the natural history of disease.

These individuals, however, do become proficient at a number of things. They learn to order all kinds of tests and procedures—but don't always know *when* to order or *how* to interpret them. They also learn to play the numbers game—treating a number or some other type of test result rather than the patient to whom the number or test result pertains. And by using so many sophisticated tests and procedures, they inevitably and unwittingly acquire a laboratory-oriented rather than a patient-oriented mindset. Contributing to this mindset, incidentally, are the health maintenance organizations that force physicians to care for a maximum *number* of patients, in a minimal *number* of minutes, for the lowest *number* of dollars.

Society's overall values and priorities are not what they used to be. When I trained in the mid-1950s, hard work, self pride, devotion to duty, strict accountability, and pursuit of excellence were the norms. Today, the emphasis is on limited work hours, on quests for personal gains, and on political correctness. Pride and (especially) accountability have mostly disappeared. As a result, people at all levels—including many medical students, house officers, and faculty members—are satisfied with mediocrity, the only norm they know.

In bypassing or curtailing the history-taking and physical examination, the high-tech approach weakens the patient-doctor bond—or prevents it from ever forming. The high-touch approach, by contrast, represents the apotheosis of Oslerian medicine, ensuring that we treat the *patient*, not the disease.

While modern medical technology has greatly enhanced our ability to diagnose and treat disease, it has also promoted laziness—especially mental laziness—among many physicians. Habitual reliance on sophisticated medical gadgetry for diagnosis prevents physicians from using the most sophisticated, intricate machine they'll ever and always have—the brain.

Is there a cure for this tyranny of technology? Any cure would be very difficult because, at a minimum, it would require a total revamping of our medical school teaching faculties. Currently, these faculties consist largely of two groups: fellows and young instructors who are fact-filled but experience-thin, and older professors who are proficient in only a narrow segment of their specialty. Both groups spend most of their time lecturing, writing papers, working in the clinics or laboratory, or traveling to meetings. These activities, whether school-decreed or self-imposed, limit contact between the faculty and trainees. And recent mandates limiting resident work hours further reduce such contact. What teaching there is takes place primarily in the lecture hall, conference room, or hallway outside the patient's room, rather than at the patient's bedside. Students and house officers end up spending more and more time attending lectures or conferences and less and less time attending their patients. With limited access to the teaching staff, the trainees turn to house officers and fellows one to two years their senior for instruction—a situation I consider "the blind leading the blind."[64]

Regardless of how we stack up in Heaven (assuming we get there), doctors *are* different from "ordinary mortals"—in two "extra-ordinary" ways. We have a license to look at, touch, or probe any part of another person's body. And we can literally bury our mistakes, typically with no outsider ever realizing that we have made them.

These differences make medicine a privileged, yet insulated, profession. If we cherish the privilege and reject the insulation, we doctors won't play God.[65]

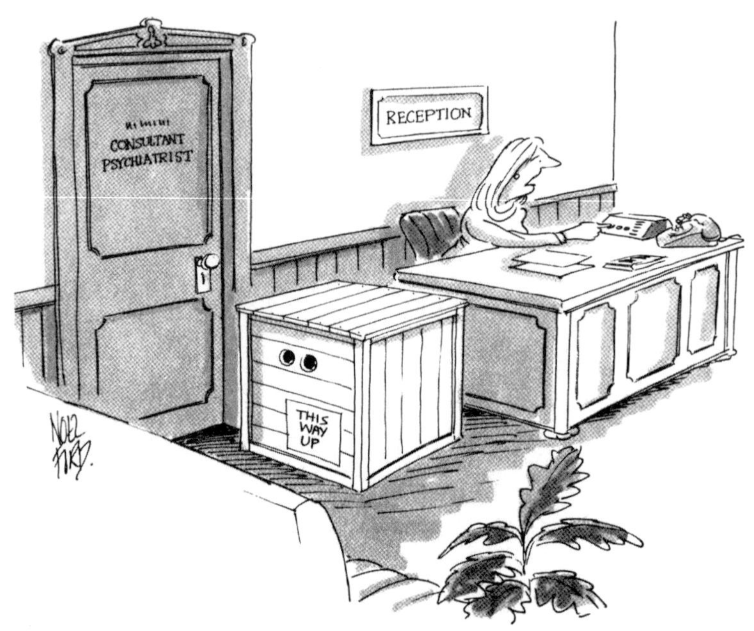

"Are you expecting a case of agoraphobia?"

Chapter Four: Herb Fred's Dictionary of Non-Differential Diagnoses

Achalasia.

On routine chest radiographs of patients with achalasia, the dilated esophagus is sometimes mistaken for mediastinal or pulmonary disease. That it may also be mistaken for cardiac disease receives virtually no mention in the medical literature, including textbooks of Cardiology, Gastroenterology, Pulmonology, and Radiology.[66]

Angiokeratoma.

The tell-tale sign of Fabry's disease is the angiokeratoma—distended capillaries protruding into a hyperkeratotic epidermis. These lesions, detectable in childhood or adolescence, appear as discrete, punctuate, purple-red papules predominantly in the "bathing suit" area.[67]

Amyloidosis.

When a patient has waxy papules on the eyelids and easily inducible bleeding, think of systemic amyloidosis.[68]

Atherosclerosis. *See Pseudoxanthoma elasticum.*

Alopecia. *See Thallium.*

Amebiasis, cutaneous.

Cutaneous amebiasis deserves consideration in any patient with extensive necrosis and ulcerations of the skin and underlying tissues. Amebic trophozoites are easy to miss in sections stained by hematoxylin and eosin; they also are easily confused with macrophages.[69]

Anemia.

Failure to examine critically the peripheral blood film of an anemic patient is a common but inexcusable error.[70]

Aortic plaque.

A chest x-ray that shows displacement of a calcified aortic plaque by 10 mm or more suggests aortic dissection. CT scanning can confirm the diagnosis if it identifies two or more channels separated by an intimal flap.[71]

Ascariasis. *See Larvae.*

Ascites.

When ascites is the first, the only, or the predominant sign of fluid retention, the doctor should administer thyroid hormone, strip the pericardium, or open the abdomen.[72]

Thyroid function studies are indicated in every patient with unexplained ascites.[72]

Ascites is a prominent early finding in constrictive pericarditis. Onset of symptoms is typically insidious, and months to years often pass before the correct diagnosis is made. Patients frequently present with decreased muscle mass, hepatomegaly, varying degrees of jaundice, and gross ascites, often with little or no peripheral edema. These findings commonly simulate those of hepatic cirrhosis or abdominal carcinomatosis. In patients with pericardial constriction, the central venous pressure is elevated and the neck veins are distended. By contrast, in patients with hepatic cirrhosis or abdominal malignancy, the central venous pressure is normal and the neck veins are flat.[73]

The *sine qua non* for diagnosing pancreatic ascites is a greatly elevated level of ascitic fluid amylase—frequently into the thousands of U/L. A leaking pancreatic pseudocyst accounts for the ascites in about two-thirds of these patients. In the remainder, disruption of the pancreatic duct is responsible.[73]

Of the curable causes of conspicuous ascites, tuberculous peritonitis is the hardest to establish or exclude. Studies from around the world show that laparoscopy or celiotomy is the best way to diagnose tuberculous peritonitis. This approach allows targeted biopsies of the peritoneum, liver, and any abnormal-appearing structure. Even if the peritoneum looks normal or merely thickened, it may still contain granulomas and should be biopsied.[73]

Asphyxia, traumatic.

Traumatic asphyxia is characterized by a striking bluish-red to bluish-black discoloration of the face, neck, and upper part of the thorax, together with massive subconjunctival hemorrhages. In most cases, the syndrome results from a severe compressive or squeezing injury to the thorax or upper abdomen. Diagnosis can be baffling if the physician is unfamiliar with this syndrome. In truth, however, there is no differential diagnosis.[74]

Botulism.

When symmetric, descending cranial nerve paralysis develops four to 14 days after an open injury and spares mental and sensory function, think of wound botulism.[75]

Bowel movements, colored.

Red-colored bowel movements can terrify the patient and sometimes mystify the doctor. The terror comes from fearing blood. The mystery comes when there is no blood. In virtually all such cases, a careful review of the patient's dietary and medication history will disclose the coloring agent. Foods known to be responsible are beets, red peppers, tomatoes, red cherries, "red hots," and breakfast cereal. Oral medications that deserve consideration include the urinary analgesic phenazopyridine hydrochloride (Pyridium®), the anthelmintic pyrvinium pamoate (Povan®), diazepam (Valium®) syrup, and rifampin (Rifadin®). Intravenous administration of sulfobromophthalein sodium (B.S.P.) to test liver function can also produce bloody-looking stools.[76]

A tarnished-silver or aluminum paint-like stool color characteristically results from biliary obstruction (white stool) combined with intestinal bleeding (black stool). Carcinoma of the ampulla of Vater is the usual cause.[77]

Cachexia.

"Cancer somewhere" all too often is diagnosed in an attempt to explain away the presence of cachexia even though many other illnesses may lead to emaciation.[70]

Cancer.

A solitary dense rib in a middle-aged or older man should always suggest osteoblastic metastasis, particularly from carcinoma of the prostate. The same finding in a woman of comparable age should suggest carcinoma of the breast.[78]

Cancer metastatic to the eyelids is rare. In nearly half of the reported cases, the primary tumor originated in the breast. The site of origin in the remaining cases has varied considerably, with the lung, skin (melanoma), and gastrointestinal system predominating.

Metastatic lid disease presents clinically in one of three ways: 1) as a solitary, nontender, uninflamed subcutaneous nodule; 2) as an ulcerative lesion; or 3) as thickening and induration of the lids. The thickened, indurated form presumably results from lymphatic obstruction by tumor cells. It occurs almost exclusively in women with breast carcinoma and occasionally is bilateral and symmetric.[79]

If a metastasis pulsates, the primary tumor is carcinoma of the kidney or thyroid gland. There are no other considerations, unless the sternum is the site of metastasis. In that instance alone, multiple myeloma is another diagnostic possibility.[80]

Catheter.

When a patient with an indwelling central venous catheter develops new or progressive cardiorespiratory distress, vascular erosion or perforation deserves immediate consideration. A lateral radiograph of the chest can be the best way to verify a malpositioned central venous catheter. Failure to recognize this complication can prove fatal.[81]

Esophagus, dilated. *See Achalasia.*

Fabry's disease. *See Angiokeratoma.*

Hookworm disease. *See Larvae.*

Hypoparathyroidism.

Seizures or papilledema or both may signal idiopathic or postoperative hypoparathyroidism. It is prudent, therefore, to obtain a serum calcium level in any patient with unexplained seizures or papilledema, particularly when carpopedal spasm or paresthesias also are present.[82]

Larvae.

Larvae in the sputum may be seen not only in overwhelming strongyloidiasis, but also in ascariasis and hookworm disease. In all three conditions, therefore, the victim may literally cough up the diagnosis.[83]

Lead poisoning. *See Red blood cells, basophilic stippling of.*

Lymphoma, conjunctival.

Conjunctival lymphoma usually occurs in persons older than 50 years and affects men and women equally. It can be unilateral or bilateral, with or without systemic involvement. The lesions typically are painless. Definitive diagnosis requires histologic examination and immunohistochemical stains of the involved tissue. Treatment consists of radiotherapy for localized disease and chemotherapy for systemic disease.[84]

Melanoma.

Malignant melanoma is the only condition known to turn a white person's entire skin absolutely black.[69]

Meningococcemia.

Meningococcemia, with or without meningitis, can be fulminating, with death occurring in less than two hours after the first symptom appears.[82]

Night sweats. *See Tuberculosis.*

Papilledema. *See Hypoparathyroidism.*

Pancreatitis.

In patients with acute pancreatitis, echymotic discoloration of the abdominal wall can occur in the loins (Turner's sign) or near the midline from the umbilicus to the symphysis pubis (Cullen's sign). These cutaneous changes, however, are not specific for pancreatitis. In the absence of trauma and blood disorders, they are merely manifestations of retroperitoneal or intra-abdominal hemorrhage.[85]

Paralysis, cranial nerve. *See Botulism.*

Pellagra.

Pellagra (*pelle agra,* rough skin) is traditionally portrayed as a niacin-deficiency disorder resulting from a diet of three Ms—meat (fatback), meal (cornmeal), and molasses—and manifesting clinically as four Ds (dermatitis, diarrhea, dementia, and death). Approximately one-fifth of pellagrins, however, manifest a fifth D—"dyssebacia"—the name coined to describe numerous plugs of inspissated sebum projecting from dilated orifices of sebaceous glands. On palpation, the plugs feel like sharkskin or sandpaper. They first appear along the alae nasi, then spread over the nose, and in advanced cases, involve the forehead, lips, and chin.[86]

Pericarditis, constrictive. *See Ascites.*

Peritonitis, tuberculous.

Multiple biopsy specimens of the peritoneum—obtained at laparoscopy or at celiotomy—are often necessary to confirm or exclude tuberculous peritonitis. [72]

Pneumonia, eosinophilic.

A chest x-ray that shows diffuse infiltrates in the periphery of both lungs, with relative sparing of the perihilar regions, is characteristic of eosinophilic pneumonia.[87]

Pseudoxanthoma elasticum.

Accelerated atherosclerosis at an early age should suggest pseudoxanthoma elasticum, especially when known risk factors are absent.[88]

Rash. *See Scabies.*

Red blood cells, basophilic stippling of.

Basophilic stippling of red cells can be the first, best, or only clue to lead poisoning.[89]

Retinal emboli.

Discovery of calcific retinal emboli should prompt attention to the heart. In many cases, the emboli stem from calcific aortic stenosis. Additional sources include calcified mitral valve or annulus, calcified myxomas or thrombi, and calcified atheromata in the aorta or carotid arteries.[90]

Scabies.

Any unexplained, persistent, intensely pruritic skin rash should be considered as scabies until proved otherwise.[91]

Sclera, icteric, unilateral.

Unilateral scleral icterus can appear under 2 circumstances: (1) the patient is jaundiced from whatever cause, and the nonicteric eye is false, or (2) the serum bilirubin is normal, and the icteric sclera reflects a resolving subconjunctival hemorrhage.[92]

Sclerae, blue.

Blue sclerae characteristically are associated with heritable disorders of connective tissue. They appear chiefly in osteogenesis imperfecta and to a lesser extent in pseudoxanthoma elasticum, Ehlers-Danlos syndrome, and Marfan's disease. Rarely, they are seen in patients with iron deficiency, rheumatoid arthritis, or myasthenia gravis. The blue discoloration occurs when thinning of the sclera allows the underlying choroid to become visible.[93]

Seizures. *See Hypoparathyroidism.*

Sickle-cell disease.

When the conjunctivas of patients with certain types of sickle-cell disease are examined with the +40 diopter lens of the ordinary ophthalmoscope, a specific alteration in the vascular pattern may be observed. The characteristic sign consists of sharply defined, dark-red, comma-shaped or corkscrew-shaped vessel fragments that appear to be isolated from the rest of the conjunctival circulation. The pathogenesis of this lesion is uncertain.[94]

Sinuses.

Most chronically draining sinuses of the face or neck have a dental origin. Because many of the patients have no dental symptoms, diagnosis may be delayed for years.[95]

Skin discoloration.

Causes of widespread bluish-gray discoloration of the skin include cyanosis, methemoglobinemia, hemochromatosis, metastatic melanoma, phenothiazine and antimalarial therapy, and exposure to bismuth, gold, or silver.[96]

Skin metastases.

Skin metastases may arise from almost any organ. They tend to appear late in the course of fatal neoplastic disease, but sometimes they are the earliest sign of cancer. The lesions usually are papulonodular, painless, discrete, and freely movable. They vary in size and number and can be easily overlooked. Biopsy is necessary for exact diagnosis.[97]

Spinal fluid, xanthochromic.

Xanthochromic spinal fluid has three basic causes: hemorrhage into the spinal canal, hyperbilirubinemia (serum total bilirubin level usually above 10 mg/dL), and cord compression blocking the flow of spinal fluid. The patient's clinical manifestations and serum bilirubin level should point immediately to the probable mechanism and to the type and extent of further workup.[82]

Strongyloidiasis. *See Larvae.*

Thallium.

Alopecia is the hallmark of thallium intoxication and develops in virtually everyone who survives the acute insult. It usually appears between the first and third week of illness, characteristically affects the scalp, and commonly spares the face, axillae, and pubic area.[98]

Tongue.

An enlarged, serrated tongue suggests amyloidosis, acromegaly, or hypothyroidism.[99]

Tuberculosis.

Despite current knowledge, many patients still undergo tests for tuberculosis just because they have night sweats. We can no longer afford this malady of practice. We should put to rest the long-ingrained notion that night sweats signify tuberculosis.[100]

Varicoceles.

Testicles don't pulsate, but varicoceles can. Pulsatile varicose veins anywhere in the body are pathognomonic of tricuspid insufficiency. The patient in question had rheumatic heart disease. (Another patient of mine had a pulsating varicocele associated with the tricuspid insufficiency of Ebstein's anomaly.)[101]

Venous stars.

The sudden appearance of venous stars on the upper chest or shoulder may be the earliest manifestation of an obstructed great thoracic vein.[102]

References

1. Fred HL. Stupid, or ignorant? Houston Medical Journal 1985;1:51.

2. Fred HL. Intellectual anorexia. South Med J 1975;68(12):1468.

3. Fred HL. Foreword, forward, four-word, or four-ward? Medical Journal of St. Joseph Hospital 1983;18:179-80.

4. Fred HL. The journey to the grave. Medical Journal of St. Joseph Hospital 1980;15:91-4.

5. Fred HL. Tenets for physicians in the new millennium. Hosp Pract (Minneap) 2000;35(2):13-6.

6. Fred HL. The sick sense syndrome. South Med J 1989;82(9):1155.

7. Fred HL. *Say Aah (Hah)! A Medical Educator Mouths Off.* Macon (GA): Mercer University Press; 1991. p. ix.

8. Fred HL. Just what the doctor ordered. Hosp Pract (Minneap) 1999;34(13):11-2.

9. Fred HL, Scheid M. I may be a fanatic, but I'm a healthy one. *USA Today.* 1984 Aug 7:12A.

10. Fred HL. What's the difference . . . And what difference does it make? South Med J 1980;73(12):1559.

11. Fred HL. On becoming a fathead. South Med J 1989;82(10):1265.

12. Fred HL. Helen. South Med J 1986;79(9):1135-6.

13. Fred HL. The Shakespearean Principle. Hosp Pract (Minneap) 1998;33(9):83-4.

14. Fred HL. Requiem for the ophthalmoscope. Hosp Pract (Off Ed) 1994;29(2):37-8.

15. Fred HL, Hassan Y. Eyeing pathogens in the peripheral blood film. Hosp Pract (Minneap) 1999;34(9):124-6.

16. Fred HL. Four-letter words. South Med J 1990;83(5):563.

17. Fred HL. As a matter of "fact". . . . South Med J 1990;83(2): 203-4.

18. Fred HL. Greasing the gut: A lesson from history. Pract Gastroenterol 2002;26(8):46,48.

19. Fred HL. Sine qua nons for the compleat physician. South Med J 1988;81(7):883-4.

20. Fred HL. These are the days: The internship revisited. Tex Heart Inst J 2007;34(1):3-5.

21. Fred HL. The downside of medical progress: The mourning of a medical dinosaur. Tex Heart Inst J 2009;36(1):4-7.

22. Fred HL. Idiopathic. South Med J 1986;79(3):351-2.

23. Fred HL. Learning medicine. South Med J 1988;81(4):422-3.

24. Fred HL. The interesting patient. Hosp Pract (Off Ed) 1993;28(4):10.

25. Fred HL. Responding to adversity: A story worth remembering. Tex Heart Inst J 2009;36(3):192-3.

26. Fred HL. Previous medical records: Lest we forget. Hosp Pract (Off Ed) 1994;29(7):79,83,87.

27. Fred HL. Dishonesty in medicine revisited. Tex Heart Inst J 2008;35(1):6-15.

28. Fred HL. On the sagging of medical professionalism. Texas Medical Board Bulletin 2004;2(Fall):1,3.

29. Fred HL. The blind leading the blind. Hosp Pract (Minneap) 2000;35(5):12,14-5.

30. Fred HL. Cause or coincidence? South Med J 1992;85(9):923.

31. Fred HL. Milton + Sutton = Mutton: "Know what to do and when to do it." Tex Heart Inst J 2009;36(4):272.

32. Fred HL. The tyranny of technology. Hosp Pract (Minneap) 1997;32(3):17-8,21.

33. Fred HL. Diagnostic derailment. South Med J 1989;82(11):1333.

34. Fred HL. Old-fashioned doctors. Hosp Pract (Minneap) 1998;33(12):15.

35. Fred HL. Remember the rattlesnake. Hosp Pract (Minneap) 1999;34(7):7-8.

36. Fred HL. Drawbacks and limitations of computed tomography: Views from a medical educator. Tex Heart Inst J 2004;31(4):345-8.

37. Fred HL. Courvoisier revisited. Houston Medicine 1992;8:65-6.

38. Fred HL. When the bell doesn't ring. Hosp Pract (Minneap) 1997;32(11):54.

39. Fred HL, Rapini RP, Jones S. Clinicopathologic conference: A black man with simultaneous multisystem disease. Houston Medicine 1990;6:161-72.

40. Fred HL. The scope of scopes. South Med J 1990;83(10):1205.

41. Fred HL. *Looking Back (and Forth): Reflections of an Old-Fashioned Doctor.* Macon (GA): Mercer University Press; 2003. p. 95.

42. Fred HL. The numbers game. Hosp Pract (Minneap) 2000;35(7):11,15-6.

43. Fred HL. Scholarly. South Med J 1988;81(7):909.

44. Fred HL. Recommended reading. Houston Medical Journal 1986;2:119-20.

45. Fred HL. ABBRS. South Med J 1987;80(11):1339.

46. Fred HL. TIA is a TIA. Houston Medicine 1989;5:76-9.

47. Fred HL, Cheng TO. Acronymesis: The exploding misuse of acronyms. Tex Heart Inst J 2003;30(4):255-7.

48. Fred HL. DLTBGYD. Hosp Pract (Minneap) 1999;34(11):15-6.

49. Fred HL. To my knowledge. South Med J 1976;69(11):1455.

50. Fred HL. Elephant medicine revisited. Tex Heart Inst J 2008;35(4):385-7.

51. Fred HL. Diagnostic and therapeutic tenesmus. South Med J 1978;71(6):617-8.

52. Fred HL. Atypical chest pain: A typical humpty dumpty coinage. Tex Heart Inst J 2009;36(5):373-4.

53. Fred HL. Doing nothing. South Med J 1992;85(4):343.

54. Fred HL. "M.D." South Med J 1978;71(8):887.

55. Fred HL. Algorithms: Let's give them back. Hosp Pract (Minneap) 2000;35(9):15-6.

56. Fred HL. Buzz words and buzz procedures. Houston Medical Journal 1986;2:42-3.

57. Fred HL. The real question. Forum Med 1979;2(9):579.

58. Fred HL, Robie P. Gimmicks. South Med J 1983;76(8):953.

59. Fred HL. The consultation: Who benefits now? South Med J 1985;78(10):1145-6.

60. Fred HL. Press box vision. J Okla State Med Assoc 1978;71(5):153.

61. Fred HL. Passing the buck. South Med J 1982;75(10):1164-5.

62. Fred HL. I remember when. South Med J 1992;85(12):1242-3.

63. Fred HL. *Elephant Medicine—and More: Musings of a Medical Educator.* Macon (GA): Mercer University Press; 1988. p. xviii.

64. Fred HL. Hyposkilla: Deficiency of clinical skills. Tex Heart Inst J 2005;32(3):255-7.

65. Fred, HL. Doctors Aren't Ordinary Mortals. South Med J 1991;84(5):550

66. Fred HL, Vaisman D, Hassan Y. Dilated esophagus mimicking cardiomegaly. Pract Gastroenterol 2002;26(1):48-9.

67. Hariharan R, Fred HL. Leg pain and kidney disease in a 38-year-old man. Hosp Pract (Minneap) 1996;31(7):119-20.

68. Fred HL. Case in point (systemic amyloidosis). Hosp Pract (Minneap) 1995;30(6):24.

69. Fred HL. *Looking Back (and Forth): Reflections of an Old-Fashioned Doctor.* Macon (GA): Mercer University Press; 2003. p. 97.

70. Fred HL, Eiband JM, Lane M. Cancer somewhere. Medical Times 1965;93(7):735-8.

71. Hariharan R, Masozera N, Fred HL. Case in point (chronic aortic dissection). Hosp Pract (Minneap) 1997;32(7):24.

72. Fred HL. Enigmatic ascites: The forgotten four. Houston Medicine 1989;5:2-5.

73. Fred HL. Curable conspicuous ascites: The forgotten four. Hosp Pract (Minneap) 1999;34(11):98-100.

74. Fred HL, Hariharan R. Sudden, persistent facial discoloration after chest trauma. Hosp Pract (Minneap) 1996;31(9):100-2.

75. Fred HL. Case in point (wound botulism). Hosp Pract (Off Ed) 1994;29(1):39.

76. Fred HL. Red or cold diarrhea: Lessons from history. Houston Medicine 1990;6:90.

77. Fred HL. A rare look at a silver stool specimen. Pract Gastroenterol 1997;21(11):44.

78. Fred HL, Hariharan R. Case in point (metastatic carcinoma of the prostate). Hosp Pract (Minneap) 1996;31(3):76.

79. Tschen LF, Tschen JA, Natelson EA, Fred HL. Photophobia and thickened eyelids in a healthy-appearing nurse. Hosp Pract (Minneap) 1996;31(2):73-4.

80. Fred HL, Salazar C, Faiz S. Pulsatile metastases: What every medical practitioner should know. Pract Gastroenterol 2002;26(10):39-40,42.

81. Fred HL, van Dijk HA. *Images of Memorable Cases: 50 Years at the Bedside.* Houston (TX): Long Tail Press/Rice University Press; 2007. p. 152.

82. Fred HL. Five cases in search of a diagnostician. Hosp Pract (Off Ed) 1993;28(4A):72,74-6.

83. O'Connor M, Fred HL. Coughing up the diagnosis. Pract Gastroenterol 2000;24(1):27.

84. Fred HL, van Dijk HA. *Images of Memorable Cases: 50 Years at the Bedside.* Houston (TX): Long Tail Press/Rice University Press; 2007. p. 84.

85. McCall RM, Fred HL. Case in point (hemorrhagic pancreatitis). Hosp Pract (Minneap) 1997;32(2):182.

86. Fred HL. "Dyssebacia"—A fifth D of pellagra. Pract Gastroenterol 2003;27(3):41-2.

87. Hariharan R, Fred HL. Case in point (eosinophilic pneumonia). Hosp Pract (Minneap) 1997;32(5):232.

88. Fred HL, Hariharan R. Hematemesis in a woman with skin, eye, and heart abnormalities. Hosp Pract (Minneap) 1995;30(9):28R,28U.

89. Fred HL, van Dijk HA. *Images of Memorable Cases: 50 Years at the Bedside.* Houston (TX): Long Tail Press/Rice University Press; 2007. p. 88.

90. Fred HL, Knight K, Hariharan R. Ophthalmoscopic and cardiac abnormalities in an asymptomatic elderly woman. Hosp Pract (Minneap) 1995;30(12):24O-24P.

91. Fred HL, van Dijk HA. *Images of Memorable Cases: 50 Years at the Bedside.* Houston (TX): Long Tail Press/Rice University Press; 2007. p. 80.

92. Fred HL. Unilateral scleral icterus. Resid Staff Physician 2004;50(11):45.

93. Fred HL. Osteogenesis imperfecta. Resid Staff Physician 2005;51(7):44.

94. Comer PB, Fred HL. Diagnosis of sickle-cell disease by ophthalmoscopic inspection of the conjunctiva. N Engl J Med 1964;271(11):544-6.

95. Fred HL. Case in point (dental sinus tract). Hosp Pract (Minneap) 1998;33(7):130.

96. Fred HL. Case in point (generalized argyria). Hosp Pract (Off Ed) 1994;29(10):14.

97. Fred HL. Undifferentiated bronchial carcinoma with skin metastases. Resid Staff Physician 2004;50(6):27.

98. Fred HL, Accad MF. Abdominal pain, leg weakness, and alopecia in a teenage boy. Hosp Pract (Minneap) 1997;32(4):69-70.

99. Fred HL. Systemic amyloidosis. Resid Staff Physician 2003:49(12):40.

100. Fred HL. Night sweats. Hosp Pract (Off Ed) 1993;28(8):88.

101. Fred HL. *Looking Back (and Forth): Reflections of an Old-Fashioned Doctor.* Macon (GA): Mercer University Press; 2003. p. 98.

102. Fred HL. Case in point (venous stars heralding carcinoma of the lung). Hosp Pract (Off Ed) 1994;29(12):16.

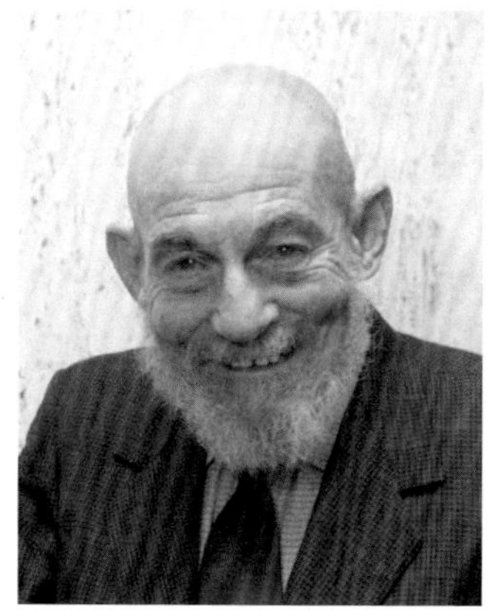

About Herb Fred

Herbert L. Fred, MD, MACP, is one of the leading medical educators and diagnosticians in America. A graduate of the Rice Institute and Johns Hopkins University School of Medicine, he has authored more than 400 publications, including 4 books. Three of his books, each a collection of provocative essays, provide philosophical insights into the practice of medicine, the challenge of difficult diagnosis, the joys, frustrations, and rewards of teaching, the pleasurable pain of learning, and the exhilaration of true scholarship. The fourth book, *Images of Memorable Cases: 50 Years at the Bedside*, was nominated for the National Book Award.

Among Herb's many honors is a Presidential Citation from President Ronald Reagan in 1988. The American College of Physicians named him its Distinguished Teacher for 2004, and gave him Mastership the same year. In 2005, he received the TIAA-CREF Distinguished Medical Educator Award. *The Herb Fred Medical Society, Inc.*, founded in 2002 by Herb's former trainees, honors him for "a half-century of bedside teaching." Many of his former students have become leaders in American medicine, including a president of the American College of Physicians, a president of a health science center, a medical school chancellor, 3 deans, 2 department chairs, 9 division chiefs, and an executive director of a state medical board.

Herb is an emeritus member of the prestigious American Osler Society, and has served on the editorial boards of numerous national medical journals. He currently is Professor of Medicine at the University of Texas Health Science Center at Houston.

In midlife, he became a runner of renown, setting numerous national age and age-group records for 50K, 100K, 100-mile, and 24-hour runs. Since 1966, he has kept a log of his daily runs, which, as of May, 2010, totaled just over 240,000 miles.

Herb lives in Houston with his wife, Judy. They have 7 children.

About Mark Scheid

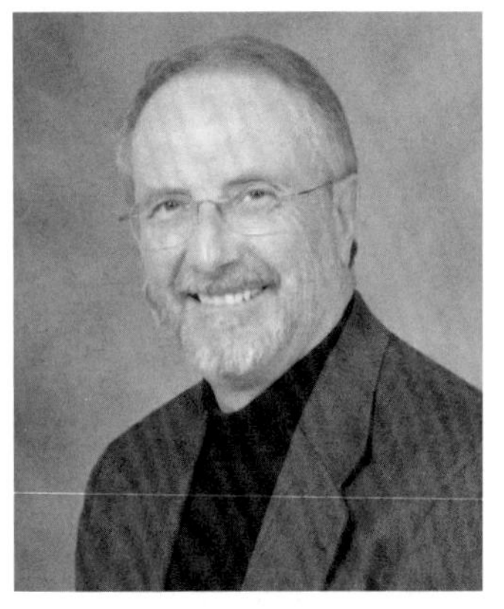

Mark Scheid is President and CEO of the Institute for Study Abroad at Butler University. From 2008 until 2010, he was President and CEO of the Tan Tao University Project in Vietnam, and served as a Fulbright Senior Specialist in higher education structure and administration, acting as consultant to a number of U.S. and international universities, most recently with a new state university in Tetovo, Macedonia.

First a professor of English, he went on to serve in the administration of Rice University as assistant vice-president for student affairs, interim vice-president for enrollment, executive director of international programs and scholarships, and assistant to the president. In July, 2008, he concluded a two-year appointment as managing director at Rice's Baker Institute of Public Policy, a period which saw the institute being named among the "top thirty" think tanks in America.

Scheid is a founding board member of the Forum on Education Abroad and an inaugural member of the Partnership Council of the School for International Training, the advisory board to the Alliance for Education Abroad and the NAFSA working group on consular and visa affairs. His most recent presentations include seminars on crisis management at several national conferences, and participation in the NSF/JSPS co-sponsored international seminars in Washington, Tokyo, and Kyoto on the internationalization of science-technology education. His latest publication is a co-authored paper on "The Georgetown University Consortium Project," the first major multi-institutional, multi-disciplinary, and multi-language evaluation of outcomes assessment among US study-abroad students.

Index